How to Lower Blood Pressure Naturally now

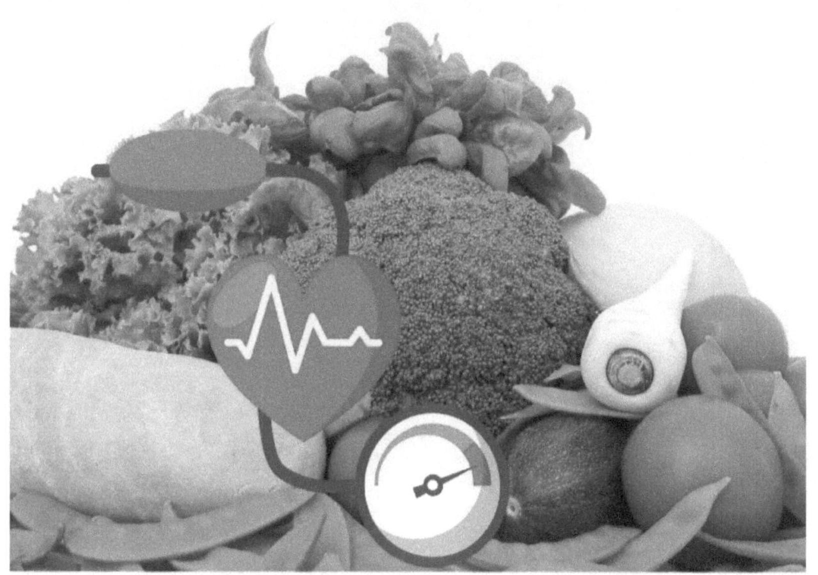

How to lower and monitor blood pressure naturally without medication

Emily Smith

All Rights Reserved © Emily Smith

All rights reserved. This book or any part of it may not be copied, edited or re-written in any format whatsoever without the permission and approval of the Author.

ISBN-10: 1661555802
ISBN-13: 979-8647429124

CONTENTS

2

Introduction

Blood pressure also known as hypertension occurs in 1 out of 3 adults in the United States and it has affected up to 1 billion people globally, investigations has shown that people die of high blood pressure daily. Lifestyle changes which is rated 70% has proven to be more effective compared to taking of medication which is 30% to lower blood pressure.

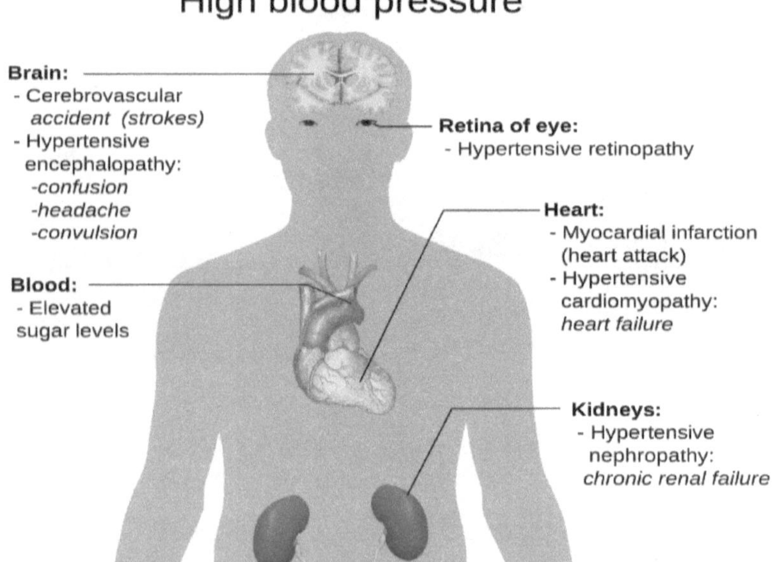

Normal blood pressure has a systolic of 120 and diastolic rate of 80 and above, it's a situation whereby blood flowing in the arteries of the heart causing a pressure on the walls of the blood vessels which is very high than normal which makes the arteries to become hardened.

There has been about 95% of hypertensive cases in the United States with one-third having it without been self-aware and most of the people with high blood pressure are between the ages of 44 to 65 and it's believed that black women having the highest incidences and there is a tendency of blacks having it twice more than whites.

There are two main types of hypertension which is essential (primary) and secondary, the first case develops mostly from childhood while you grow into an adult and the secondary is caused by another disease in the body such as kidney disease, apnea, thyroid, adrenal gland tumors, natural congenital in blood vessels, medications and illegal drugs such as amphetamines and cocaine.

High blood pressure also known as a "silent killer" can be in your body system for long without you knowing it, so it will good to carry out a H.B.P test once in a while to make sure you keep your body healthy.

Though there are few symptoms some people do experience in there body such as nose bleeding, headache, breathing shortness, nausea, dizziness, chest pain, abdominal pain and this symptoms are only noticed when it has reached an advanced stage.

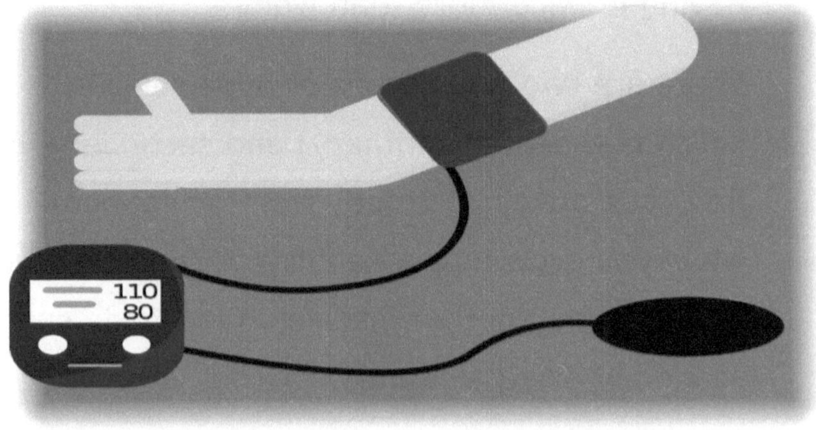

Medical specialist have always advised that on people who are from 18 years old and above should at least visit the hospital for high blood checkup in every 2 years while (18-39-40) years should go for checkup yearly even if they haven't noticed any symptoms or health issue relating to hypertension.

 Because it's possible it to be developing in your body as your growing older. It has some certain measurement levels examples.

Normal is less 120/80 mm hg

Prehypertension 120-139/ 80-89 mm hg

Stage 1: 140-159/90-99

Stage 2: 160/100 above mm hg above

It's measured using a sphygmomanometer which was replace with mercury devices.

Visit a doctor when you observe it keeps going higher.

When you don't pay attention to high blood pressure due to your busy schedules it may cause you some serious health risk with time such as heart attack, kidney failure, stroke and loss of vision etc.

In this book you're going to be introduced to unique ways you can lower your blood pressure and keep on working on it for the rest of your life to remain healthy and avoid sudden health challenges as a result of high blood pressure.

 I promised you will surely learn something new in this book which will help to improve on your current high blood pressure situation.

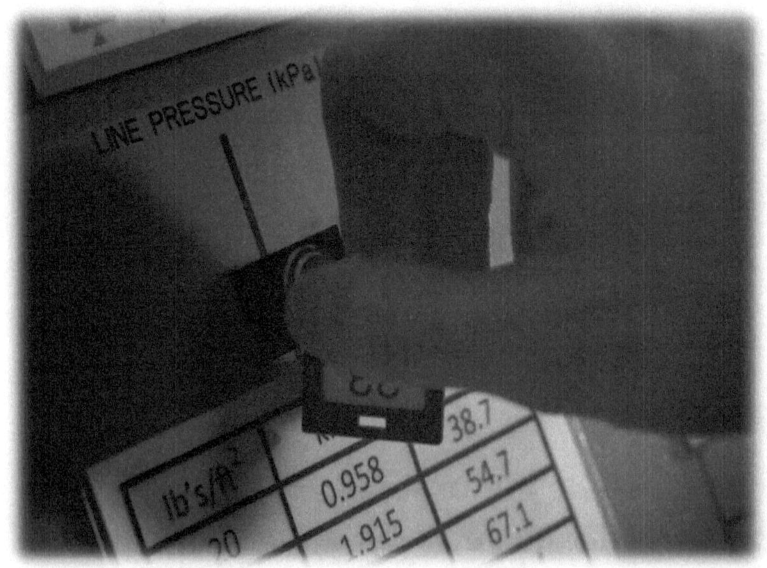

High blood pressure causes

There are no specific known symptoms of high blood pressure that's why it's referred to as "silent killer" and when it's very high it contributes to other health issues such as;

- Memory loss
- Vision loss
- Dementia
- Metabolic syndrome
- Heart failure
- Kidney failure
- Stroke
- Heart attack
- Aneurysm

Risk factors that cause H.B.P

Age Above 35 years

Family history

Race

Obesity

Inactive

Pregnancy

Kidney disease

Diabetes

Sleep apnea

Birth control pills

Excessive alcohol

Smoking

Poor diet

Effective exercises that lower B.P

When High blood pressure is chronic, it then becomes a very serious health challenge and it has no permanent cure yet, but there are things you can do to lower it down to maintain a good and healthy lifestyle and also not resulting to other health issues.

There are numerous exercises recommended but we have selected few that we fill are more effective to write on so that you can be properly informed and carry them out from time to time when free to lower high blood pressure.

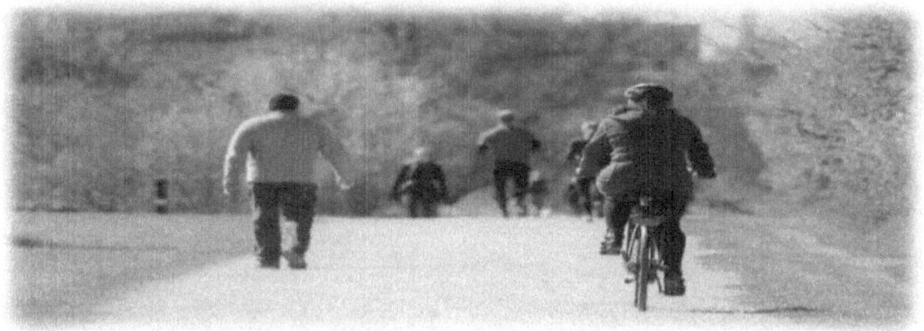

Walking; it's a natural way of bring down high blood pressure that has proven to be very effective and if you're a very busy person who is always at school, office or work place you can take few minutes of your break to do them, let's say, like 10 minutes each for a little walk around and get back.

It's advisable for you to walk at least 30 minutes daily for effective performance, you can wear fitbit to monitor the time you spent and known your heart beat rate, and if you do it constantly in few months' time you will discover positive changes in your body system.

However there are two types of walking the light walk which is just a strolling and brisk walking which is more intense and it's the recommended type which will actually get your heart pumping blood very well.

I will advise you to always carry out brisk walking for you to get better results faster, Walking is very important and sometimes it's recommend you start workouts even before going to see your doctor for checkup and measuring it because it exercises the heart directly.

Riding bike; morning bike riding can help on your cardiovascular health allot because cycling helps in strengthen your leg muscles, pump blood effectively around the body and can reduce blood pressure up to 10mm hg.

Cycling is an aerobic exercise that deals extensively on muscle training, it's believed that stationary bike cycling helps even more to regulate blood flow in body muscles and you can be doing it every few minutes each day and on weekly basis. If you have more time you do it always for better and faster result and get a heart rate monitor to be observing your heart beat rate.

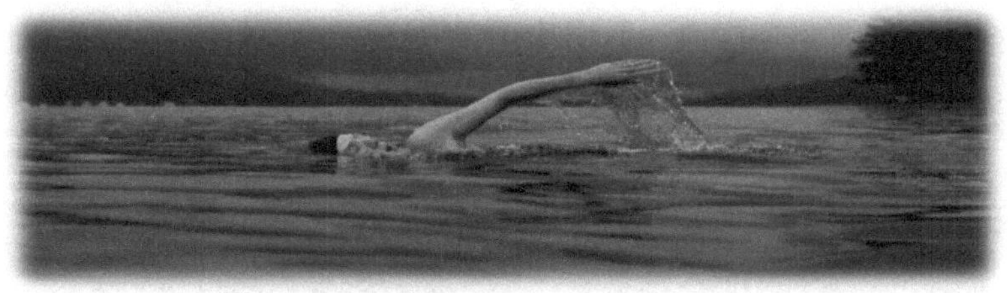

Swimming; swimming is considered to be very effective especially in older people due to overheating of joints caused by other exercises and water buoyancy is very good for joints and ankles.

Swimming has been known to reduce the systolic level which is the top measurement of blood pressure drastically in less than few weeks or months if you take some few minutes or hours to swim daily and the process of taken a dip in the pool to swim is also recommended because it helps to lower blood pressure better.

Jogging and running; Are endurance cardiovascular exercises which are also good for the body muscles, they are highly intense for the body so with that your heart will pump blood very well, so it will nice of you to take some time out to be doing them always and you will start seeing positive results.

But in case of any chest pain or dizziness you should stop immediately and see your doctor.

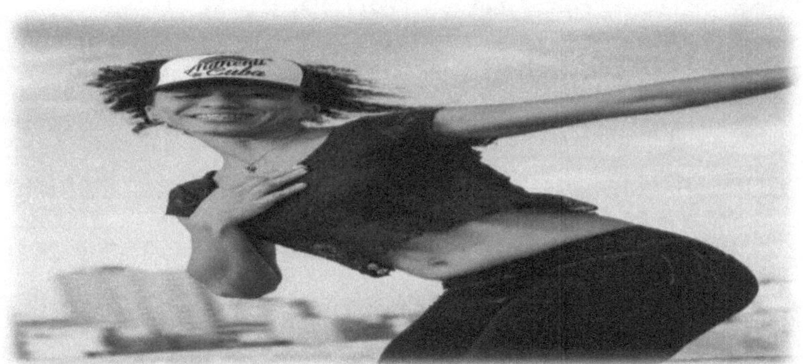

Dancing; it's a fun way of reducing high blood pressure which involves swaying your body muscles interchangeably which has shown to reduce high blood pressure at an alarming rate.

It helps reduces stress and weight as well and make blood flow in the body in a that will lower the level of blood pressure, there are recommended dance styles to help you lose weight easily such as samba, salsa and hip-hop.

Reducing stress

There are stress hormones such as cortisol and adrenaline which affects your body negatively due to working yourself tirelessly on daily basis and not taking a break so it's one of the factors that has been contributing to high blood pressure as a result of being stressed all the time without rest.

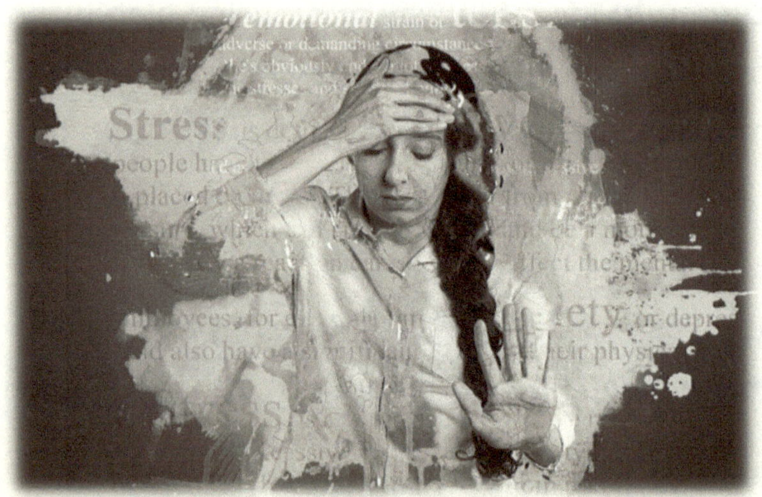

These are some of things you need to take into consideration so that you can work on them regularly to reduce high blood pressure in your body system.

Sleeping; Sleeping properly and on time helps in relieving your body from stress and when you wake up it will become fully active and functioning and blood flow will also be regulated and lower blood pressure.

Practice relaxing; there are techniques that can help you relax such as yoga, meditation etc., which involves progressive muscle relaxing with stress busters, taking a deep breath will also relieve your nerves which are always stressed to be relaxed.

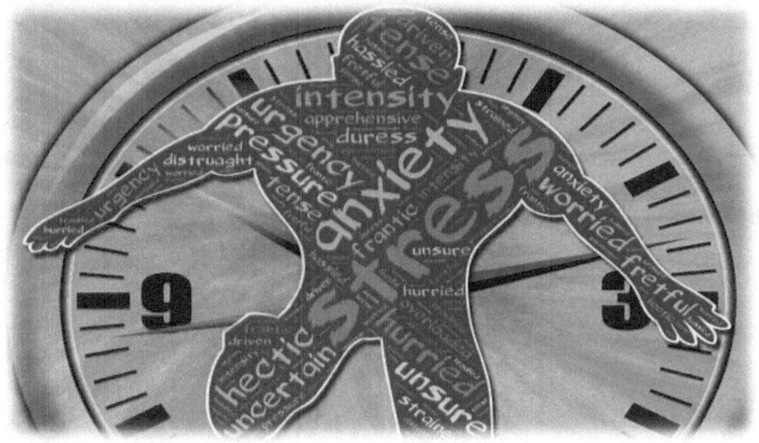

Talking to friends; chatting or sharing your high blood pressure problem with friends who have more ideas on things that you can do that will help you reduce stress is encouraged.

Because some of them might have been through same issues in the past and they found solutions on it and so they can advise you perfectly on what to do and steps to follow.

Body care; There are daily things that you need to do constantly to reduce stress such as eating of healthy foods, worrying less about issues beyond your control, exercising always so that you can be physically fit to be able to lower high blood pressure.

Schedule; have a do-list to plan out your daily activities so that you can be able to figure out the more stressful ones to reduce them then re-schedule them when the weather is friendly so that it won't stress you much, let's say try doing them when the weather is less harsh like morning, evenings and not doing in afternoon.

Reducing sodium intake

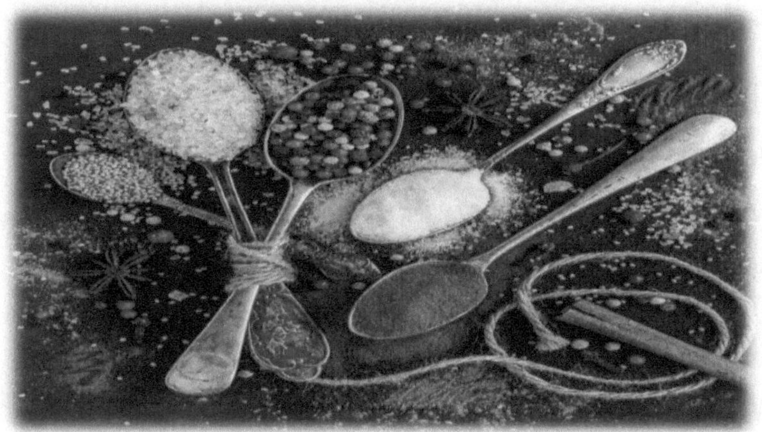

SOdium which is found in salt is believed to be one among the causes of high blood pressure with 75% of it being in processed and packaged foods, so most H.B.P patients are advised to make their own food themselves so that they can be able to add the quantity of salt they want as recommended by a doctor.

The United States federal guideline for sodium intake for adult is 2,300 mg or less but people still people do take up to 3400 mg of sodium, medical evidence has proven that reduction of sodium will lower high blood pressure and other disease such as stroke.

There are ways you can cut down sodium intake such as looking at food labels before you purchase for consumption, canned foods such as tuna, vegetables and beans should be properly rinsed before cooking.

When cooking it's advised that you add spice to your meal in replacement for salt such as parsley, black pepper, coriander, ginger, garlic, onion powder, dry mustard, thyme, cumin, nutmeg, marjoram, cilantro etc.

There are precautions you need to take into consideration as you go about your daily activities such as buying packaged or processed foods with lower-sodium, when in a restaurant make sure you know the quantity of salt added to any meal before eating.

When eating in your house try to avoid reaching out to salt shakers on the table and if you can't avoid it, then stop eating at the dining table if you can't resist it, since you can't stop eating processed foods make sure you take little quantity of it always to avoid accumulation of sodium in your body system.

Generally eating too much salt has some negative effects apart from causing high blood pressure, you will always be having swelling of legs, experiencing shortness of breath and overall body discomfort each time.

When you have a kidney disease, too much salt will lead to fluid retention and it will also contribute to weight gain and bloating as well.

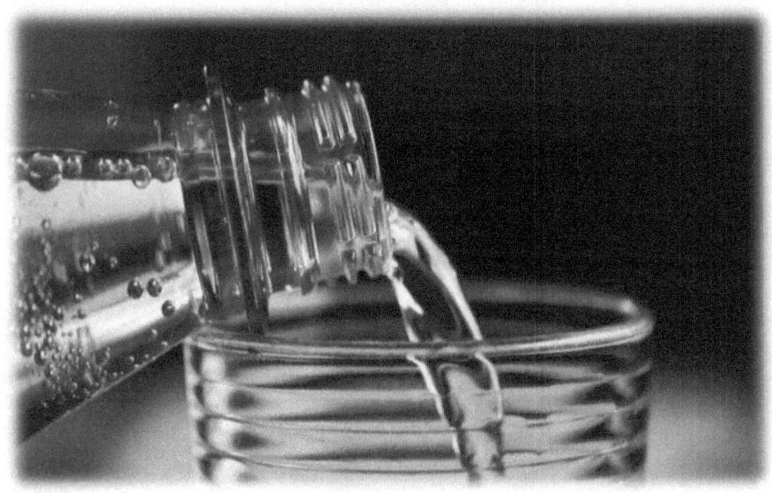

There is also risk of complications from diabetic patients, so there are other ways you can reduce salt intake but less effective based on investigation.

Drinking a specific quantity of water to wash out salt in the body system, and then sweating it out with the use of high intense exercises that will make you sweat allot.

There is 500 mg of salt in a pound of sweat and it's recommended that you use a sea-salt in replacement for table salt.

<u>Reducing alcohol Intake</u>

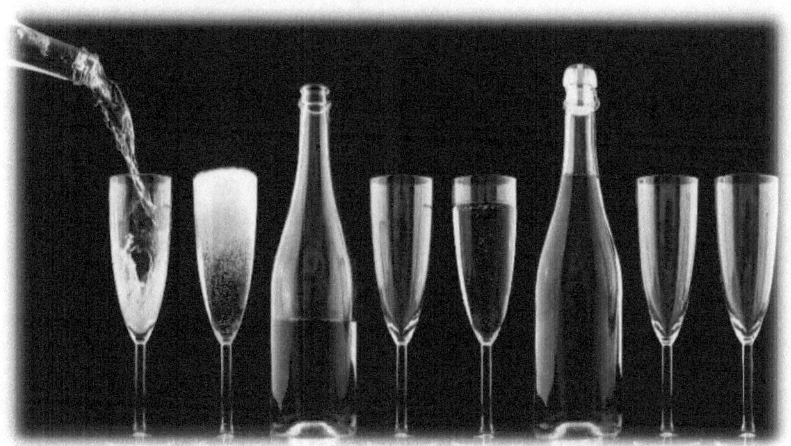

Alcohol is known to have allot of calories, therefore drinking too much of it will make you gain allot of weight and from there your blood pressure level will increase.

There are recommended guidelines for men, women and adults to specifically consume at least 14 units weekly so that you can take it moderately you will be able to control its intake and there won't be a high blood pressure.

 There is a recommendation for people of all ages and it's as follows;

Men below 65 years (should take two drinks a day)

Men older than 65 years (should take one drink a day)

Women of any age (should take less than one drink a day)

There has been a case of heavy drinkers who stopped drinking and suddenly developed high blood pressure, so it's advisable to start the process gradually let's say from daily, weekly there you can start adding more until you gradually reduce it to a barest minimum and finally stop.

Tips on reducing Alcohol

Spacers; it's a trick whereby when the urge to drink comes, you simply substitute it with beverage drinks that are mostly nonalcoholic and sometimes little alcohol in them such as soda or juice and drink plenty of water with the little alcoholic beverage drinks.

Triggers; there are certain friends, places and activities you need to distance yourself from so that you won't be triggered to start having an urge to drink so that you can't resist and decide to take little quantity and from there you will take much, but it was because you were with a drinking friend or a drinking joint.

Make a list or diary; make sure you write down the quantity you want to drink in a day, weekly and monthly to know if you're actually progressing on reducing your quantity intake.

And try to involve alcohol free days in your list and from there you can decide to test yourself by going off alcohol for some few days to see if you can cope.

Peer pressure; learn to have the strong mind to say no for a drink when given in any environment you find yourself which can be on friendly visit, inside someone's office, an occasion or anywhere you find yourself and don't kind keep alcohol at home anymore if not you will tempted to drink when you see it.

Substitute Habit; one of the surest ways of reducing or stopping a bad habit especially an addiction to prevent health issues such as high blood pressure, it's recommend that you look for something to substitute with drinking alcohol.

You can substitute it with a sport or activity in such a way that when the urge to drink comes you can go out to do it and spend allot of hours there and when you come back you won't even fill like drinking anymore, repeat this things for days and weeks and you suddenly realized it will become your new habit.

Consistency; to achieve any goal in life one has to be consistent, making sure you take the rules of rejecting alcohol, calculating what quantity you drink, not keep it at home and staying away from people or places that will trigger you to drink.

<u>Dash diet</u>

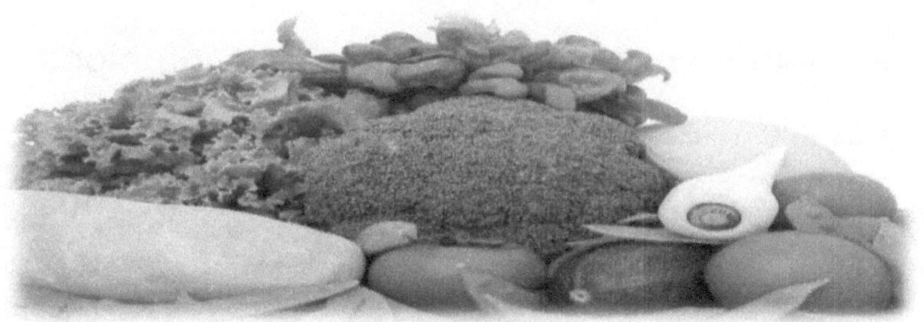

Dash which stands for dietary approaches for stopping hypertension, it's an approach designed for eating in a healthy way so that you can lower high blood pressure, it was designed as a substitute for medication by the national health institute and some physicians.

It emphasizes on fruits, whole-grains, vegetables, and low-fat or fat-free dairy products, poultry, fish, nuts, beans and vegetable oils.

It's advisable that you limit some certain foods that are highly saturated with fat such as full-fat diary with its products, fatty meats, tropic oils such as palm oils, palm kernel and coconut oils coupled with sugar-sweetened sweets and beverages.

The dash diet can help you reduce high blood pressure with few points in a week or two, the systolic which is on top of measurement can reduce 8 to 14 points which is a very significant difference when we talk of health risk for lower blood pressure.

There are two types

Standard dash diet; consumption of 2,300 mg of sodium daily.

Lower sodium dash diet; consumption of 1,500mg of sodium daily.

Dash diet eating plan;

- **Fruits;** they are mostly fiber, contains potassium, magnesium and are free from fats except coconut.
- **Vegetables;** carrots, sweet potatoes, tomatoes broccoli and most vegetables are made up of fiber.

- **Low fat or fat free dairy foods;** cheese, yogurt, milk and most dairy products are made of vitamin D, protein and calcium.

- **Lean meats, fish and poultry;** it's good you cut back on meat so that your meal will have more vegetables, because meat contains protein, iron, zinc and vitamin B.

- **Grains;** they are mostly found in cereal, pasta, rice and bread.

- **Nuts, dry beans and seeds;** types of foods here are kidney beans, peas, lentils, almonds and sunflower and they contain protein, magnesium and potassium.

- **fats and oils;** fats are essential for the body absorption of vitamins and immune system but when they are too much in the body you risk having diabetes, obesity and heart disease. Examples are mayonnaise, dressing salad and soft margarine, Dash diet assist in reduce 30% of fat calories daily.

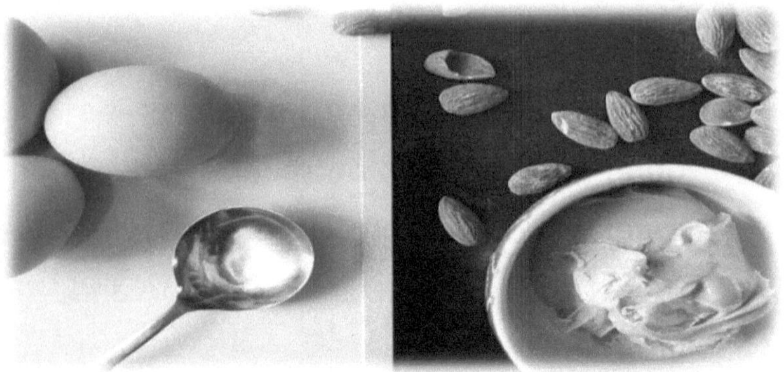

Examples on how to apply them to meals.

- **Fruits :4 to 5 servings**

One medium pc of fruit

63ml ¼ cup of dry fruit

125ml ½ of fresh, canned / frozen fruit

- **Vegetables: 4 to 5 servings**

250ml One cup of leafy raw vegetables

125ml ½ cup of vegetables cooked

- **Low fat or fat free dairy foods: 2 to 3 servings**

250ml one cup of milk

50g one and half Oz of cheese

250ml one cup of yogurt

- **Lean meats, fish and poultry**

  3 ounces of lean meats cooked

  Fish or poultry without skin

- **Grains:7 to 8 servings**

  One bread sliced

  250ml one cup of cereal to eat

  125ml ½ cup of pasta, cooked rice or cereal

- **Nuts, dry beans and seeds:4 to 5 servings**

  1/3 cup of nut (1.5oz)

  ½ cup of peas and cooked dry beans

  2 tea spoon ½ Oz seeds

  30ml 2 tea spoon of peanut butter

- **fats and oils:2 to 3 servings**

  30ml 2 tea spoon of light dressing salad

  5ml 1 tea spoon of soft margarine

  5ml 1 tea spoon of vegetable oil

  15ml 1 tea spoon mayonnaise low-fat.

Natural remedies

There are natural fruits, spices and herbs which without medication has proven over time to help reduce high blood pressure naturally apart from diet and other natural forms of activities.

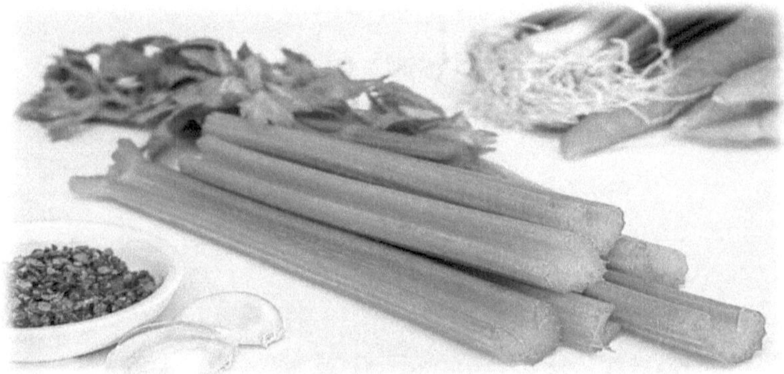

Celery; it's a Chinese cultural seed used to lower high blood pressure, a fibrous vegetable that serves as a diuretic which is responsible for flushing water that is excess from the human heart.

This singular act lowers blood pressure, the seeds are usually inserted into drinks, tea and cooked meals and it should be added 3 times daily.

Sesame oil; this seed oil have omega-6s polyunsaturated fatty acid, (sesamin)a lignin compound of sesame oil has proven to be effective in lowering blood pressure, and vitamin E.

They are all good when it comes to lowering blood pressure, diabetes and cardiovascular diseases in the body, lignin makes sure cholesterol absorption is reduced in our body, Sesamin and (PUFA) relaxes arterial wall together and lower high blood pressure and 1 ounce of oil or sesame seed should be added to meals at least for 2 months.

Cayenne pepper (capsaicin); well known as a vasodilator, it expands blood vessels quickly and there will be improved blood flow in our body which then pressure is taking off faster on arteries and blood pressure reduced.

Capsaicin is an ingredient in red pepper, when pepper is more Spicer then it means it contains more capsaicin which is responsible for creating newly red cells of blood and with improvement in blood structure, also aids with the detoxing of blood and plaque build-up removal from arterial walls.

It reduces bleeding faster when you're injured so make sure you sprinkle it on the wound properly. And when using it add just 1 teaspoon daily and gradually increase to 2-3 teaspoon daily.

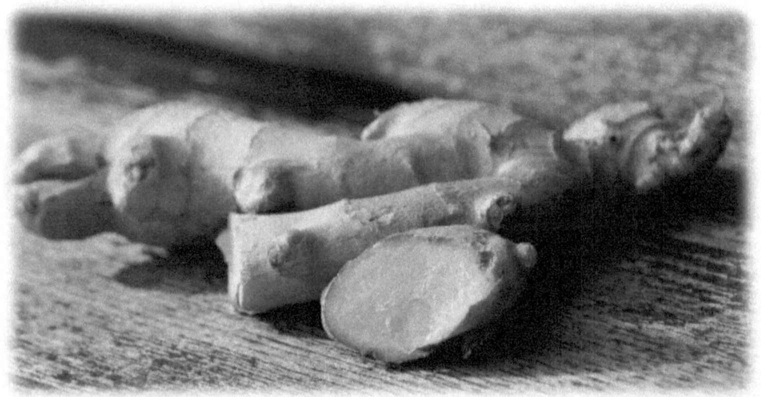

Ginger; it has been known for a very long time for healthy benefits in our body system for heart issues and reducing blood pressure, blood clot prevention and cholesterol.

It's a blood thinner for reducing clotting of blood so that you won't have stroke or heart attack, so make sure you add it to juices and smoothies in your meals daily.

Garlic; it's very popular when it comes to lowering blood pressure, A herb that helps with blood thinning compounds with an improvement in cardiac health conditions.

A diuretic that naturally forces out sodium that is excess inside our body with water and send it to urine and blood pressure is reduced most especially from a heart that has been over worked.

It can be mixed 1 or 2 mince cloves into cup, add water, shake and then drink.

Cardamom; it's a spice mostly used in Ayurveda medicine, it's also used for respiratory disorders, renal issues, gastrointestinal disorders, heart burn and cardiac disorders, cardamom is an antioxidant, antibacterial, anti-cancer properties, gastro-protective and anti-spasmodic.

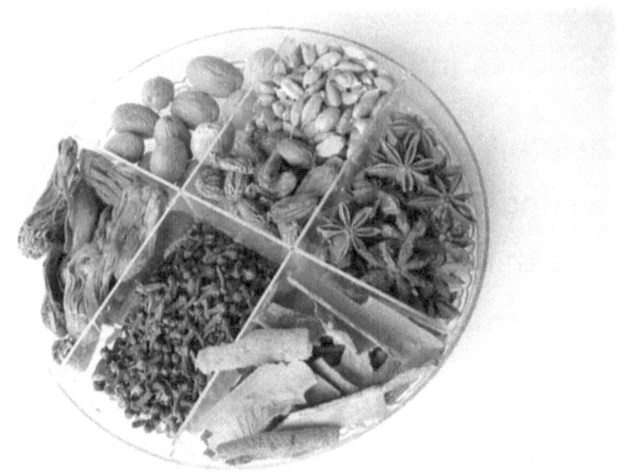

It causes blood vessel dilation and blood flows easily and it's pressure is reduced, so 1 teaspoon of mix cardamom powder with organic raw honey poured in a cup of filtered warm water and it should be taken 2 times daily.

Mistletoe; it's normally beautify so you may not have a slight taught it can be used for lowering blood pressure in your body system, but known to boost your immune system, treat hepatitis, cancer and lower blood pressure.

Its extract has a compound that is active known as alkaloids, which are responsible for lowering high blood pressure with nerve impulses controlled around the heart and arterial walls.

Mistletoe doesn't work very fast in the body but it can have a long lasting positive effect on your body when it comes to reducing blood pressure.

Though it can be poisonous and harmful if eating in a raw or unprocessed form, so talk to your health specialist before making use of mistletoe extract to prevent hypotension.

Carrots; they have allot of antioxidants called beta-carotene, vitamin C and A which lower free radicals causing cancer in your body system which is also responsible for preventing damage of blood vessels with cellular death.

They are high in potassium and electrolyte, potassium makes sure the fluid in our body system balances and stabilizes and lower blood pressure because it opposes sodium in our body which has negative effect with its excess quantity.

It's advisable to make carrot juice and drink 1-3 cup daily, but it should be organic with no added sugar.

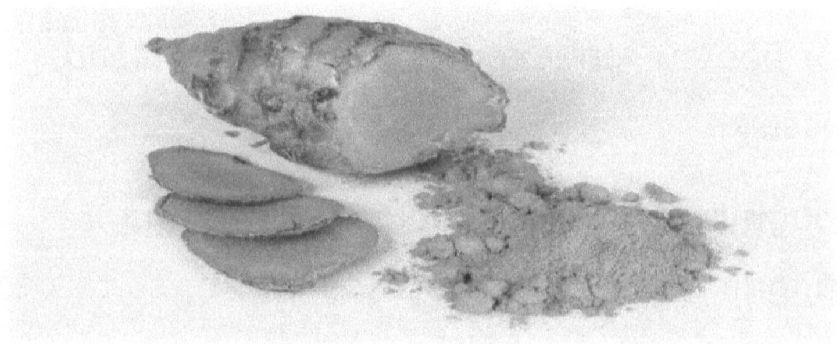

Turmeric (cur cumin); it's a spice known for inflammation decrease in the body and improvement of the flow of blood and helps in cardiovascular function, it removes plaque build-up on arterial walls.

It's also a blood thinner which helps in lowering blood pressure, turmeric powder should be included in tea with ginger and organic honey, and it's also available in capsules.

Cat's claw; a popular Chinese herb, in central and south America it's mostly used for the treatment of blood pressure with the help of inducing vasodilation and blood will flow easily in the body, it's also a diuretic and has flavanols and tannins which give out a chemical called nitric oxide(NO).

It keeps vessels open and vital oxygen with nutrients are able to circulate in the body system and dilate vessels of blood which reduces body stress and therefore lower blood pressure, a dose of it is 350 mg and should be taking daily.

Potassium intake

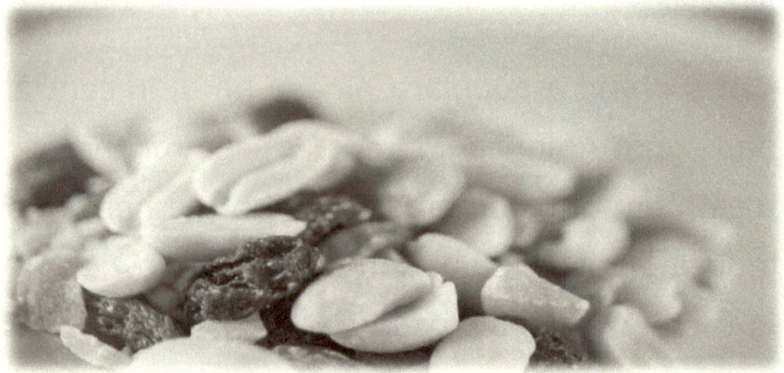

Potassium intake has proven to be very effective when it comes to reducing of sodium in our meals, both potassium and sodium are similar in chemical formation so potassium takes the sodium out of the cell while it goes in and this helps our cells to function very well and for our body energy production as well.

Package foods are the main sources of sodium intake, so avoiding them greatly will potentially reduce your sodium intake as it's known that 2% less of Americans achieve a balanced recommendation for potassium intake which is supposed to be 4,700mg per day.

There are certain foods which are very rich in potassium and as someone who has high blood pressure you are advised to start consuming them serious to improve your health condition.

List of potassium rich foods.

- Spinach
- Lima beans
- Tuna
- Potatoes
- Raisins
- Peas
- Tomato juice and sauce
- Mushrooms
- Halibut
- Molasses
- Berries
- Apricots and it's juice
- Avocadoes
- Grapefruit and it's juice
- Prunes and it's juice
- Fat-free yoghurt
- Cantaloupe and melon of honey dew.

<u>Quit smoking</u>

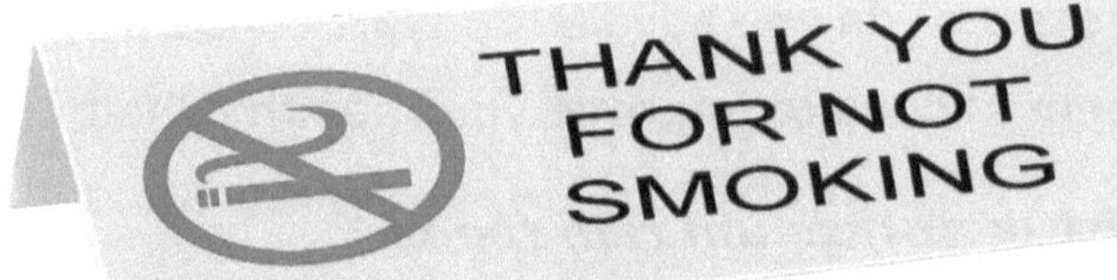

Smoking cessation is a something anyone with very high blood pressure issue needs to take into serious consideration and then gradually stopping it because the negative effect of it in your body is diverse as it affects your body system.

There is nicotine that is contained in each cigarettes which usually raises heart beat rate and cause high blood pressure with arteries being narrowed, hardening of its walls, clotting of your blood and stress which will lead to stroke or heart attack.

There are ways of reducing smoking gradually until you can stop, because like every other addiction you can't just stop it suddenly in the middle of the day, you need constant practice on how to gradually reduce it and be persistent and you will see positive results.

It's believed that alcohol or drinks with caffeine can trigger you to smoke, so the best way to stay off it is to also reduce alcohol intake gradually.

When the urge to smoke comes you can suppress it with low-calories foods like carrot, sugar free candies and sugar free gum.

Keep away from joints or friends with serious smoking habits for your own good, if truly you are serious about smoking cessation and it's advisable you take a deep breath and then exhales and smoking urge will pass and you will continue with what you were doing.

Most effective ways of stopping any addiction is replacing that habit with a similar healthier type, so you can get nicotine gum or patches and chew when the urge comes.

Weight loss secrets

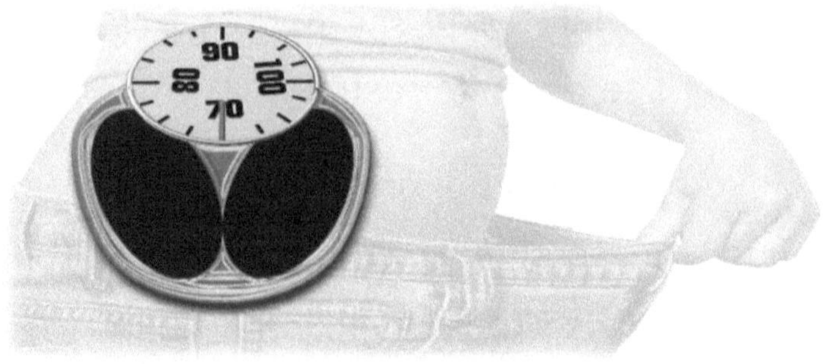

Weight gain and obesity are caused by food and drinks which built up calories in our body system through daily consumption of drinks and foods, so when the body has taken in excess of energy.

It stores it in the body as fat and it will into make you gain weight, therefore it will be good for you to change your eating habits to lose weight.

When you change the foods you have been eating which made you to gain weight you will consume less calories and you will start seeing changes on your body weight, most especially foods like snacks contribute so much in building up calories in your body system, so it will be good for you to start avoiding foods with allot of sugar as they also make you gain weight.

There are certain things you need to do on a daily basis to lose weight such as exercising regularly for faster and better results.

You can also get heart health cookbooks online to know more about diets that lower blood pressure so that you can be doing them, also learn deep breathing techniques to help you relax and relieve your body of stress.

When exercising its good for you to always check your blood pressure so that from there you can know if you are having positive results, make sure to take the treatment plan your doctor prescribe for you seriously.

Naturally losing of weight has been proven to work effectively with exercises than any form of weight reduction anybody tells you so stick to exercises and your weight will reduce.

Secret lowering tips

Lifestyle changes; change of activities in your life can be a great way to help you lower your blood pressure if you can't keep up with regular exercise and constant medications and its believe that lifestyle changes works very well and some doctors have confirmed that it's even better than medication if you take your new lifestyle changes seriously and maintain it.

There are issues that if you truly know you can't handle just let go so that they won't be on your mind and as a result of thinking about it cause your blood pressure to rise.

Try to be comfortable with the level of your life at present and live a happy life, laugh, joke and gist, also spend some time with your family, listen to classical music and eat good meals to relax your nerve then your body will be relieved and there will be normal blood flow within the body system.

Reduce too much luxury even if you are wealthy, try to walk to nearby places to like 30 minutes every day of the week to see someone or purchase something.

Avoid things that will triggers you such as "rush-hour" so that you will not start rushing and panicking that you're late to.school or work, because such things leads to high blood pressure.

House chores are also activities you can do to regulate good flow of blood in your system when your free at home you can cut flowers, clean dirt within your courtyard, cleaning and washing etc.

This activities makes you active and therefore regulate normal blood flow in the body, because being one place makes you to be inactive and it can contribute to high blood pressure. It's also good to sit in the sun once in a while for few minutes so that it can boost chemicals in the body that makes you feel good which are known as endorphin.

Conclusion

Blood pressure is a universal health issue which all human are faced with time as life goes on due to our daily lifestyle which we all live and when you start having this health challenge.

It will become part of your life so it will become a long term commitment for you to constantly look after your body system to learn and practice ways of lowering it so that you can leave a normal life.

High blood pressure mostly occur in people between the ages of 35 and above but since it happens to everyone with time, it's good for you to start monitoring your body even before you get to the age 18 for you to start going for test once or twice in a year due to its silent nature.

There are natural ways of reducing it such as exercises, switching habits, dash diet, and daily precautionary measures to reduce stress, reducing alcohol, sodium intake and aerobics that provide better results than medication, so it's advisable you start doing them before you can even go and see a doctor for checkup and test for further diagnosis.

There are allot of things you need to reduce to lower high blood pressure that you should take serious if you really want to see positive results and become healthy again with blood regulating properly in your body system.

There are addictive habit you have been doing over the years which have been affecting your health and causing your blood pressure level to increase.

At this stage of your life you need to stick to recommended ways of eating meals, exercises and change of lifestyle by substituting them for other healthy issues meals and drinks such as taking beverage drinks in place of alcohol and constant exercises and activities to lower high blood pressure naturally.

ABOUT THE AUTHOR

Emily smith

A Writer, researcher, online publisher and digital content marketer who has researched and written so many books on health and fitness niche with 5 years of experience.

Disclaimer

Information or content in this book should not be used as a substitute for professional medical advice or for any medical, treatment or diagnosis, it's only meant for information purposes only, please consult your personal doctor for professional advice. Thank you.